Strategies For Dealing With Emotional Eating Outside Your Home

Strategies For Planning Home Meals: Planning, Organizing, And Implementing

Elliot Harvey

TABLE OF CONTENTS

CHAPTER ONE: STRATEGIES FOR PLANNING HOME MEALS. 3

CHAPTER TWO: HOW TO BURN FAT AUTOMATICALLY AND FEEL FULLER ON LESS 21

CHAPTER THREE: ARRANGING TRIPS TO THE SUPERMARKET ... 36

CHAPTER FOUR - PLANNING, ORGANIZING, AND IMPLEMENTING 53

CHAPTER FIVE: EATING OUT, STRATEGIES FOR DEALING WITH EMOTIONAL EATING OUTSIDE YOUR HOME 71

CONCLUSION 110

CHAPTER ONE: STRATEGIES FOR PLANNING HOME MEALS.

Earlier in the book, I talked about emotional eating and the disorders associated with emotional eating. Go through those points, and you'll notice that it is so simple to have a kitchen loaded up with intentional and healthy decisions to assist you with keeping on track with your healthy diet program. As a part of my expert practice, I visited numerous homes. Because of what I have seen and what a large number of my customers have let me know, I accept that a great many people who have attacked their eating systems need to address revamping their kitchen—and I'm not looking at placing in new machines or counters. I mean, they have to accommodate what food they keep in their homes with how they store it and how they control it.

EFFECTIVE WAYS FOR PLANNING YOUR HOME MEALS

You can control your home food condition by devising a couple of basic procedures—and here and there, this undertaking involves association and arranging. When you are feeling extraordinary and inspired, here are a few procedures that may help food redesigns in your home:

- Only purchase the food in small portions as you need.

If you purchase more food than you can use within a brief time, solidify it, share with other individuals, offer it to a food bank, part with it, or even toss it out. You may think about what a loss to dispose of food. However, is it extremely a deal if enormous food purchase is exchanged for excess weight in your body? At what expense? Are you exchanging your food abundances for your wellbeing, your association with yourself, your association with your loved ones, or with your activity?

- Place things that entice you, and you accept that you have to have close by in a territory hard to get to. For instance: If you have a subsequent ice chest, put the thing far away or put the thing high in a cabinet where it is hard to reach —Place enticing food in a storage room you don't utilize and see constantly.

- When treats and tidbits entice you, choose to permit yourself a humble serving and set the rest away. For instance, if potato chips or confections are an exceptional treat for you, partition some into a little bowl and, before you devour the treat, set the fixed sack away in an inaccessible, difficult to arrive at the pantry. Have a list dependent on your arrangement for the whole week! Record it.
- Shop after you have eaten. When you are hungry, everything looks great, and you will perpetually fill your shopping basket with hasty purchases.
- Shop the dividers to buy, however much entire and new foods as could reasonably be expected. The greater part of your new things is along the edge of the store, for example, milk and dairy, leafy foods, grains, and meats. A portion of the things in the passageways are hazardous because they contain handled food, snacks, high-fat, and fatty treats.

- Watch out for displays of specials or new foods that are, for the most part, at the parts of the bargains. These presentations are in your face deliberately, and organizations pay truckloads of money to be in your face!
- When it goes to those powerful specials in tempting displays or in food coupons—ask yourself, "Is it extremely a deal If I don't have it on my list and it's not part of my program?"
- Know the areas where you are easily attracted to food. Write in your Journal and survey the segment on "Most loved foods that push me into excess weight gain," and audit your systems for keeping away from those difficult foods.
- Pick who you go out with to the supermarket to shop with. A few people who go with you can undermine your best expectations: kids who need sugary treats, family members who have various thoughts regarding what you ought to and shouldn't eat, and good-natured Friends who may have an effect on your shopping rehearses.

- Read names if you are picking bundled or handled foods. (See what you should search for in the following segment on perusing food names.) As a savvy, key customer, state to your self, "I will...":
- Plan ahead for a seven day stretch of food needs and make a composed basic food item list.
- Shop after you have eaten.
- Shop the dividers to buy new foods; however much as could be expected.
- Read the names when you have to buy bundled or prepared foods.
- Stick to my list.

• Leave the kids at home, if possible, so there is less impulse to purchase outside of my list.

- Abstain from going shopping for food with somebody who could attack my arrangement.
- Purchase just those things on my list and abstain from utilizing coupons since I have them for different things, not on my list.

- Avoid spur of the moment purchases and promoting ploys to make such buys.
- Shop with a help individual, or If I should shop alone, be sure that I will adhere to my arrangement.

CAREFULLY READ FOOD LABELS

When you read food labels, you are searching for a lot of sugars, fats, fiber, or sodium in the list of ingredients. Essentially, you have to know a couple more things about reading food names to guarantee that you're getting the entire picture. The first ingredient recorded is the most important arranged by weight; the last fixing recorded has a minimal sum in an amount in the specific item. Additives and flavorings should likewise be recorded.

Sugars: Names for sugar are glucose, sorbitol, sucrose, dextrose, lactose, xylitol, etc. Different types of sugars include corn sugar, unadulterated sweetener, darker sugar, crude sugar, mannitol, corn sugar, corn syrups, sorghum, molasses, and nectar. There are various distinctive fake sugars available today. New fake sugars are springing up in food items all the time. The best way to remain careful is to eat everything with some restraint.

Fats: Components in many of the foods we eat are soaked in fats, including oils, grease, suet, shortening, and spread. Soaked fats are additionally found in meats, for example, hamburger, and other creature items, for example, egg yolks, spread, cheddar, sharp cream, and all milk aside from skim. Palm and coconut oils are likewise soaked fats. Unsaturated or Polyunsaturated fats are found in fish and plant foods, for example, avocados, nuts, seeds, olives, and oils, for example, sunflower, soy, nut, and canola oils. Mono-saturated fats are olive oil and rapeseed oil. Omega 3 unsaturated fats are found in sleek fish, for example, salmon, and mackerel.

Trans-fats, which means fluid vegetable oils that have been transformed into strong fats by hydrogenation, are found in margarine, many snack foods, heated products, and seared food. The words hydrogenated or halfway hydrogenated methods trans-fats are in the food—generally prepared food sources. Fats are frequently used to make mayonnaise sauces, flavors, and a plate of mixed greens dressings. Different names for fat are mono-glycerides, diglycerides, triglycerides, lecithin, lipids, egg yolk, and mayonnaise.

Salt: A mineral fundamentally made out of sodium chloride, salt is basic for most creature life. It is one of the fundamental tastes and is utilized as a significant additive. Salt is found in ingredients records for ocean salt, kelp, heating powder, preparing pop, monosodium glutamate, sodium saccharin, sodium nitrate, sodium propionate, and anything with sodium in its name. Sauces, flavors, plate of mixed greens dressings, onion salt, garlic salt, celery salt, canned tomato items, ketchup, bean stew sauces, grill sauces,

Worcestershire sauce, cooking wines, escapades, miso, hydrolyzed vegetable protein, yeast, arranged mustards, soya sauce, tamarin, pickles, corned meat, handled items and cheeses can be high in sodium. A general rule is to constrain your admission of foods that contain more than one mg — sodium per calorie. Foods guaranteeing "low-salt" or "no-salt" on their marks are best—however, read the name to ensure the case is valid. Fiber: Diets are improved with fiber. Dietary fiber originates from plants and isn't processed in the intestinal tract yet might be used in the lower gut.

Various plants have various types of fiber: gelatin and gum (which are water solvent), and adhesive, cellulose, hemicellulose, and lignin (which are water-insoluble). Wellsprings of dietary strands are discovered distinctly in plant foods—for instance: entire wheat, entire grains, oat wheat, multi-grain, rye, oats, dark colored rice, wild rice, entire grain pasta, crisp foods grown from the ground, plates of mixed greens, beans, lentils, split peas, nuts, seeds, and dried products of the soil considerably more. They aid absorption and guaranteeing that the stomach and digestion tracts function admirably. In marking, the fiber substance of food is recorded in weight just as a level of the day by day admission esteem. Also, here's the last word on shopping for food: If you need somebody to buy staple goods for you since you feel that you are excessively occupied or accept that being in a market is unreasonably enticing for you at the present time — proceed.

Keep in mind this is about YOUR success, and success implies loving and taking care of yourself. When you are more certain about your capacity to the basic food item shop, return to your list of strategies that you feel are significant for you to pursue and go complete it.

FAMILY MEALS

Our general public is portrayed by busy people from every walk of life. We are occupied individuals in our business and in our private lives. Family life can be as entangled as it is occupied, as we attempt to be all over and everything for the remainder of our relatives. Our youngsters are the ones who will endure the most If they never realize what it feels like to have sound, formal dinners with discussion and family. Family suppers ought to be solid in sustenance—for the soul and mind just as the body. You can serve scrumptious dinners that are brisk, nutritious, and engaging for the whole family.

There are numerous sources to assist you with structuring and plan healthy family dinners: cookbooks, magazines, the web, and unique media programs. From these sources, you will find food organization and cooking methods that are lower in fat, sugar, and sodium. While there are great deals of pre-arranged sound foods at the supermarket that can be served rapidly for your benefit, there are many inexpensive food dinners you can make at home utilizing entire foods. For instance, look at certain plans in cookbooks for diabetics, low-fat cookbooks, or heart-savvy cookbooks for solid supper plans. Explore them all and, the majority of all: plan, plan, plan!.

If being too occupied is your major challenge, there are a few procedures that can help conquer time-challenging weeks. For instance, be imaginative and amass freezer suppers on Sunday before the week begins. Have an assortment of dinners prepared for whatever state of mind strikes you and your family. Everybody could have something other than what's expected if they like. You can make cooler dinners that are sound and fun, as well. For all suppers, however, particularly family dinners, it is ideal to take a seat at the table to eat as opposed to eating in your vehicle or before the TV. The standard here is to slow down!

Set aside some effort to visit with the family, talk about the day, and put your fork or knife down if food is in your mouth. Bite your food as opposed to breathing in it! Appreciate each snack and taste the food! If the family demands foods that you know are unmistakably not in your eating plan and you have a test with them, you may settle on a decision to remain in charge by eating your principle supper previously or after the family eats. While they eat, you can have a plate of mixed greens. Along these lines, you are not enticed by their decisions are as yet at the table for discussion and participating in the family gathering. You realize what will work for you.

Make an arrangement early. If you don't feel great getting ready family dinners, request support from your family for some assistance. You may be astounded what they think of. The perfect, obviously, is to plan foods you would appreciate that are nutritious and a good time for your entire family. One father told me that he was not very good at arranging dinners and continued putting it off. He additionally said that his teenaged little girl was always delighted in preparing meals, so I proposed that he let his little girl plan the suppers for the week, and he could double-check them for taste and satisfaction. His food organizing challenge was understood.

Food preparation can be one of the absolute most noteworthy factors in making healthy meals. Be aware of food preparation descriptions, for example, deep-frying, coated, or adding of fat/oil to cook. These techniques include a bigger number of calories and fat than it is vital. Better strategies for planning healthy meals include grilling, baking, steaming, boiling, broiling, microwaving, barbecuing, roasting, poaching, braising, and stir-frying.

Here are a few tips to reduce the fat, sodium, and sugar in your cooking:

- Drain off the fat that collects during cooking.
- Refrigerate sauces, soups or stews, and flavors before serving so as to skim off the hardened fat that has ascended to the top. Warm them.
- In planning meats, cut back off excess as much at conceivable and expel the skin from poultry before cooking.

- When you pan sear, utilize a low-sodium stock instead of oil to cook meats and vegetables. To thicken sauces, use cornstarch or rice flour.
- In some preparing supplant fats with fruit purée or no-fat yogurt fitting for the formula.
- Reduce the measure of sugar or salt in a recipe.
- Reduce the measure of cheddar in the recipe (low-fat obviously).
- Avoid cooking your vegetable dishes with fat and salt, or including fat and salt at the table.
- Use all the crisper garlic, onions, peppers, or new herbs in your dishes.
- Add a dash of flavor to your preparation; decrease the sugar, and include vanilla or almond concentrates or cinnamon powder for the season.

Snacks

Snacks are a significant piece of family dinners, whether they are eaten at home or while away. Organized and laid out in your kitchen, custom made snacks and tidbits have a few benefits.

When taken to class or work, they frequently free us from the stress of what we will have for lunch and questions regarding how to remain on our eating plan. Other than being savvy, pre-made snacks fend off us from enticing and normally less nutritious cheap food and eatery suppers. We know precisely what is in our pre-made snacks and can incorporate the best possible adjusts for ideal sustenance and good dieting. Assortment in lunch and snack foods isn't an issue since we can bundle and convey hot and cold food sources. Scraps frequently make amazing snacks. Utilize a canteen for hot or cold foods; warm sacks and little cooler packs can guarantee freshness. Making snacks and bites at home takes effective planning.

Plan ahead for seven days of snacks and lunch that will cater to the entire family. Set a suitable time for collecting snacks sacks ahead of time—for certain families, the prior night functions admirably, and for other people, the morning appears to be less difficult. I plan my lunch and snacks for my days off as well; then, when I'm getting things done, I realize I can adhere to my eating plan.

Put variety and nutrient-filled ingredients in every one of the snacks, keeping desserts, carbonated beverages, sodium, and fats to the base or disposing of all together. If you need recommendations, ask your family, different guardians, or search for information on lunch proposals on the web. If you are enticed to snacking on the ingredients as you set up the lunch meals, request that other relatives assist you with making them. If you are eating at home, pursue similar standards for all family dinners: sit together, take part in the discussion, put down your utensils between chomps, bite completely, and turn off telephones, radios, and TV interruptions. Make the most of your time together over lunch!

CHAPTER TWO: HOW TO BURN FAT AUTOMATICALLY AND FEEL FULLER ON LESS

In this chapter, you're going to figure out how to reduce your size, become healthier, and feel full even when you're eating less food. Utilizing the simple and straightforward nutrition rules stated in this section, you'll effectively accomplish your ideal weight, and it won't appear as though you're on an eating regimen. In fact, you don't need to starve yourself or surrender your preferred foods. You'll likewise have no issue keeping up your new body shape since you're not going to do anything strange or extraordinary to achieve it.

Losing fats on your body doesn't rely upon fat grams, sugar grams, feast timing, food blends, macronutrient proportions, singular micronutrients, or any of a hundred other extraordinary diet program subjects. None of those matters in case you're eating excessively. At last, almost every weight reduction system returns full-cycle to whether it encourages you keeps up a calorie deficit. Remaining in a calorie shortage reliably, be that as it may, is a challenge on the grounds that such huge numbers of factors impact the amount you eat and what number of calories you consume.

Energy balance is dynamic, which implies the measure of calories you require can change. Alongside thinking little of food utilization, neglecting to alter your calorie consumption when your vitality needs change is the most widely recognized reason for weight reduction levels. The central issue is, "What is the most effortless, proficient, and most beneficial approach to keep up that imperative caloric shortfall?" For my cash, I'll wager on what I call "high-low" food, a way to deal with food determination dependent on three significant standards:

1. Energy density, otherwise called calorie density, is the number of calories in a portion of food for every serving.

2. Nutrient density is the dietary benefit per serving (nutrients, minerals, phytonutrients, and fiber).

3. Satiety is defined by how full a portion of food or dinner makes you feel and how that influences the amount you eat. To boost fat loss while enhancing your wellbeing, you will likely pick foods that contain the most noteworthy supplement density, the highest satiety level, and the least calorie density.

Is a Calorie, "Just a Calorie?" You might be thinking, "There's significantly more to nutrition than just calories, and a calorie isn't only a calorie!" That is the general purpose of eating nutrient-dense, normal foods. Clearly, 200 calories from pretzels and soft drinks won't give the equivalent dietary benefit or satiety as 200 calories of broccoli and salmon. Various foods can significantly influence your wellbeing, your hormones, and even your disposition, sharpness, and mental work.

Various kinds of foods can likewise have marginally various consequences for body structure at a similar gross caloric consumption. This can be clarified by the thermic impact of food, calories in stringy foods that aren't totally assimilated, and the impact of food on hormones and consequent craving. In any case, this doesn't negate the calorie law; it checks it. Representing every one of these components, when you take a look at the net outcome, you're left with precisely what the math directs: weight changes depend on calories in versus calories out.

From a vitality balance perspective, a metabolizable calorie is only a calorie. There's a major distinction between "don't count calories" and "calories don't count." Some diet regimen programs discourage calorie counting; they basically show you what to eat and what not to eat. The exceptional food blends or remarkable topic of the diet regimen is generally credited for the weight reduction. What they don't let you know is that their eating rules cause you to eat less consequently.

A DIFFERENT DEFINITION OF COUNTING CALORIES

At this point, you might be thinking, "God help us, not another calorie-counting program!" If so, take a deep breath. You won't need to check calories until the end of time.

Truth be told, in case you're determined about not including anything, I won't demand it. I'll essentially request that you complete three things:

1. Recognize the calories-in versus calories-out equation.

2. Know about your bit sizes.

3. Increase or reduce your portions in light of your week by week results.

My definition of checking calories may not be what you think. Checking calories doesn't need to mean strolling around with a scratch pad or electronic gadget, recording each piece you eat consistently. Rather, you make a day by day menu plan as your eating objective for the afternoon. Utilizing this strategy, you possibly need to tally calories once when you make your menu.

This technique is proactive, not responsive. You record what you intend to eat first, then eat it, as opposed to eating first and afterward recording what you just ate. Consider it menu arranging as opposed to calorie checking. To counteract weariness and get a dietary variety, you can make various menus or make food substitutions from a similar class with comparable caloric qualities. Making your very own menus is simpler than you might suspect. Basically, pursue the ten Body Fat Solution food rules, and your menus will nearly make themselves.

CALORIES 101: ASCERTAIN YOUR DAILY MAINTENANCE CALORIES

One size doesn't fit all with regards to calories. It's senseless to endorse a similar measure of calories for everybody, particularly If it bumps people or dynamic and inactive individuals together. For instance, 1,500 calories daily may be ideal for most ladies to reduce fat; however, it could be semi-starvation for a gigantic and active man. The greater and increasingly dynamic you are, the more calories you have to keep up your weight. Keep in mind these focuses and that both can change. Likewise, remember that ladies are commonly littler than men, so ladies, for the most part, need around 600 to 800 fewer calories every day. Calorie needs likewise decline as you get more established. As indicated by exercise physiologists Victor Katch and Frank McArdle, the normal female between the ages of twenty-three and fifty has a calorie maintenance level of around 2,000 to 2,100 calories for each day and the normal male around 2,700 to 2,900 calories.

CALORIES 102: MAKE THE ALL-SIGNIFICANT CALORIE DEFICIT

To shed fat, you should make a caloric deficit. A caloric deficit, otherwise called negative energy balance, implies that the quantity of calories you devour is not exactly the number of calories you consume. You can make a shortage by diminishing your food admission, expanding your movement level, or both. If you require 2,800 calories for each day to keep up your weight and you eat 3,300 calories every day, you're in positive energy balance by 500 calories, and you'll put on weight.

If you eat 2,300 calories every day, you're in negative energy balance, and you'll get thinner. A caloric shortfall is basic subtraction. To figure your optimal caloric admission for diminishing muscle to fat ratio, subtract 20–30 percent from your support level. 20% is viewed as a preservationist shortage; 30 percent, a forceful shortfall. In case you're a normal male, and your support level is 2,800 calories for each day, then a 20 percent shortage is a 560-calorie decrease, which gives you an objective of 2,240 calories for every day. In case you're a normal female, and your upkeep level is 2,100 calories for each day, then a 20 percent shortage is 1,680 calories for each day.

It's commonly best to keep your calorie decrease preservationist from the outset. In case you're not getting the pace of fat misfortune you need, you can make a progressively forceful shortfall later by diminishing your calories a little further or expanding your movement. Overall, most ladies will decrease muscle to fat ratio adequately and securely on 1,400 to 1,800 calories for every day. Most men will accomplish healthy, safe, and effective fat reduction around 2,100 to 2,500 calories each day. Keep in mind that these are midpoints. If your body is huge and you're dynamic, utilize the upper end of these ranges. If your body is small in size or if you're inert, utilize the lower end of these ranges.

CALORIES 103: MODIFY YOUR CALORIE INTAKE OR EXERCISE OUTPUT ON THE BASIS OF YOUR RESULTS

There are numerous equations you can use to ascertain your calorie needs with accurate precision. In any case, don't be excessively worried about calorie calculations, since you'll need to modify your calories dependent on your week after week results in any case. All you need is a decent pattern. At last, it's progressively significant that you comprehend the 10,000-foot view of energy balance. Despite the number of calories you believe you're eating at the present time, if your body weight isn't changing, then you don't have a calorie shortfall. This implies one of three things:

1. You thought little of what number of calories you are eating.

2. You overestimated what number of calories you are consuming.

3. Both of the above-mentioned. Whatever the explanation, you have to make or restore a shortage by eating less or practicing more.

THE SELECTIVE REDUCTION OF CALORIES

There are two different ways to make a shortfall: increment your vitality use or decrease your food utilization. On the food decrease side, the following inquiry is, "Which food sources do you cut?" Do you basically eat somewhat less of everything? That would work because any caloric deficiency will cause weight reduction. In any case, there's a superior way.

At that point, when a reduction in calories is called for, you specifically decrease the calorie-density basic sugars, dull carbs, and grains. That leaves the fundamental proteins, fats, and micronutrients from products of the soil moderately immaculate. If the calories fall too low to even think about satisfying your vitality needs, you essentially include caloric counterbalance by somewhat expanding your lean protein and solid fats. In case you're an insightful reader, you may be thinking, "Hello, hold up a moment, aren't you making another low-carb diet in a mask?" Well, yes and no. Truly, on the grounds that we're expanding your caloric shortfall by diminishing certain carbs. No, because there are some significant contrasts in my methodology contrasted with "conventional" low-carb abstains from food:

To start with, this diet plan isn't an outrageous low-carb diet. It's a moderate-carb sustenance program. Second, the measure of carbs you decrease isn't fixed; it's a variable dependent on your needs and inclinations. Third, the sort of carbs you wipe out directly from the beginning are the prepared carbs, refined sugars, and man-made carbs.

As results manage, you additionally lessen normal starches and grains, which are calorie thick. There's no motivation to evacuate high-nutrient density foods like leafy foods. Fourth, the essential center isn't around carbs, yet where it ought to be — on the calories. Conventional low-carb slimming down mindset can some of the time lead to the misconception and judgment of alive and well and nutritious foods and makes carbs resemble the reason for heftiness. The reason for weight isn't carbs; it's an overabundance of calories, an abatement in physical activity, and every one of the components that lead to this vitality irregularity.

The Macronutrients:

Protein, Carbohydrates, and Fat Like calories, the correct admission of the three macronutrients—proteins, solid carbs, and fundamental fats—is basic. Be that as it may, If you essentially pursue the ten Body Fat Solution food runs, your macronutrient needs will be met, and you'll naturally be in the ballpark with every one of your numbers. What's most significant is to get the fundamentals first and locate a restorative macronutrient balance that keeps away from the boundaries. From that point, you can alter the arrangement to address your issues. Before we proceed onward to the ten principles, how about we quickly review the three macronutrients. The Power of "protein" originates from the Greek word proteos, which signifies "of first significance." This is fitting since when you set up a feast, I need you to consider lean protein first. Consider protein building material for the body on the grounds that the amino acids in protein are utilized as development material for almost every cell and tissue, including muscle. Protein is found in numerous foods, even vegetables, beans, vegetables, and entire grains. While this is significant for veggie lovers to know, when we allude to "lean proteins" in this program, we're alluding fundamentally to the lean wellsprings of complete proteins, ones that contain all the basic amino acids. Complete proteins incorporate chicken bosom, turkey bosom, lean red meat, fish, shellfish, egg whites, and low-or nonfat dairy items.

Protein assumes some significant jobs in weight control. Slender protein encourages you to keep up your fit weight when your calories are confined. It additionally smothers your craving. Eating lean protein expands your digestion because of the thermic impact of food, which is how a lot of vitality you consume to process the food. Protein has a thermic impact of 30 percent. This implies If you eat a lean protein food that has 100 calories, 30 of those calories are utilized to process and process the food, leaving just 70 calories of net vitality accessible. Sugars have a thermic impact of 10–15 percent, while dietary fat has the least thermic impact of just 3 percent. A significant research survey distributed in the Journal of the American College of Nutrition briefly summarized the intensity of protein.

CHAPTER THREE: ARRANGING TRIPS TO THE SUPERMARKET

Dietitians gauge that 40 percent of store purchases are made on motivation. Now and then, you'll need to examine food marks at the store to settle on the better decision between two things, yet the entirety of your significant purchasing choices ought to be made ahead of time. Follow my shopping tips underneath, and you'll turn out each time with low-calorie, high food that draws you nearer to your objectives. Ensure you shop from a list.

Shopping records are anything but difficult to make by utilizing everyday menu designs and including the provisions required for seven days of menus. When you have your list, stay with it. As indicated by New York University sustenance teacher Marion Nestle, 70 percent of customers carry records into the grocery store, however just around 10 percent stick to them.

- Try not to shop when hungry. I'm certain you've heard this counsel previously, yet do you heed to it?
- Never shop on an unfilled stomach.
- Be aware of your physical and emotional state, also.
- In case you're worn out or upset, you're bound to snatch low quality food on motivation.
- Shop rapidly. Did you realize that general stores play downtempo music to impact you to shop all the more gradually? It's valid. If you wait for longer, you purchase more. Rather, with list close by, perceive how quick you can hurdle through the store. It helps if you shop during off-top hours when there are no groups and shorter lines.
- Do the greater part of your shopping in the aisles of the store. 80% of the foods you'll need to eat all the time can be found on the outskirts of the store: natural products, vegetables, servings of mixed greens, potatoes, yams, lean

meats, fish, fish, dairy items, and eggs. Be careful with food item promotion. In each square inch of the store, you're being advertised to always. Food organizations pay for prime areas on the racks.

- Watch out for craving animating colors, for example, red, orange, and yellow are utilized to cause you to notice snack foods. Adhere to your arrangement and don't be taken in by promoting, including wellbeing and weight reduction claims. Eat generally foods with one fixing and no name. 80% of the foods you eat every day will come without a mark (think products of the soil).
- If they have a mark, they'll normally have just a single fixing, as on account of lean meats, fish, eggs, or antiquated cereal.
- Become a specialist at checking the names.
- Prior to eating anything in a crate, can, or bundle read the mark cautiously.

- Reduce the quantity of white flour or any refined sugars, for example, sucrose or high-fructose corn syrup, are high on the list.

Do likewise if the ingredients incorporate trans-unsaturated fats or synthetic substances with names you can't articulate. Additionally, observe the calories, serving size, and fiber sum. Watch for name escape clauses. As indicated by food naming laws, if there's not exactly a large portion of a gram of fat, the mark can say "fat-free." If there are less than five calories for every serving, the name can say "zero calories." Food organizations exploit these escape clauses by contracting their serving sizes. For instance, a run of the mill non-stick cooking shower will say "calorie-free" on the name, yet cooking splash is 100 percent oil. How would they pull off it? The serving size is a 33%-of-a-second shower. Oppose drive buys at the register. Indeed, even as you're looking at, regardless, you're being showcased too. Pretty much every checkout path has treats and soft drink inside arm's compass.

Shop for food supplies on the web. A study distributed in the International Journal of Behavioral Nutrition and Physical Activity found that individuals on fat-misfortune programs who requested their staple goods utilizing on the web conveyance administrations bought 28 percent less calorie-thick foods than individuals who shopped in the grocery store.

ANTICIPATING RESTAURANT EATING

If there's one huge error that is bound to disrupt your program than some other, it's making awful decisions at cafés. In many investigations, eating every now and again in eateries corresponds to the higher muscle to fat ratio. Everything bodes well when you take a look at how things have changed in the previous quite a few years. In 1955, Americans burned through 19 percent of their food spending plan on dinners arranged outside the home. Today that number has dramatically increased to 41 percent.

The quantity of individuals now overweight has dramatically increased with it. Stoutness has significantly increased. As indicated by the U.S. Branch of Agriculture, $222 billion is gone through consistently at cafés and $118 billion of that at drive-thru eateries. The huge issue: unhealthy dinners, to a limited extent, because of expanding segment sizes. Numerous ordinary café suppers contain 1,000 calories or more in principle course alone. If you incorporate a tidbit and treat, that could include at least 1,000. One cut of cheesecake for pastry can interfere with you 700 calories. Cheddar nachos or seared mozzarella sticks have around 800 calories. The "ordinary" servings that are. As indicated by a report in Men's Health magazine, the most noticeably awful nachos checked in at 2,740 calories. A run of the mill steak house prime rib or porterhouse could without much of a stretch fall in the 1,200-to 1,500-calorie extend. Suppose you had hors d'oeuvres, fries, sweet, and beverages with that. The National Restaurant Association reports that the normal individual eats out 4.2 times each week. With that recurrence, If you picked any of these "calorie bombs" each time you ate out, it would totally undermine each nutritious handcrafted supper you ate and all that you did in the rec center throughout the entire week.

Obviously, I understand that telling individuals they can't eat in cafés won't make me extremely well known, so my progressively moderate idea is essentially to downplay eatery eating. One of the qualities I've found in most of the lean individuals is that they like to keep more tightly command over their wholesome admission by making their very own large portion suppers. If the national normal is four café dinners for every week and you don't need a normal individual's body, then don't do what normal individuals do. Do what lean individuals do. Keep eating at the cafe a few times for each week and settle on the correct decisions when you're there. Notwithstanding how regularly you feast out, you need to instruct yourself about the healthy benefit of eatery food and have an arrangement in advance.

- Start with low-calorie plates of mixed greens rather than fatty hors d'oeuvres.
- Stay away from broiled foods, for example, French fries, onion rings, and calamari.
- Inquire as to whether you don't know how something is readied, particularly about additional sauces, oil, spread, or other shrouded calories.
- Look into menus and calorie information on the web and settle on a sound decision ahead of time.
- If you don't have the foggiest idea of what number of calories are in a dish, don't eat it.
- Pick broiled chicken or fish for lean protein. Pick lean sirloins or filets and get nine-to twelve-ounce cuts or littler.
- Request steamed vegetables as side dishes.
- Request dry heated potatoes, sweet potatoes, or darker rice as sides or part of the primary course.
- Request a crisp natural product for dessert.
- Split a customary sweet with a friend.
- Try not to wipe off your plate—take a doggie pack home with you.

- Eat just until you are 80 percent full.
- Never stuff yourself.
- Try not to eat at buffets.

PLANNING YOUR WEEKENDS

Unless your Saturdays and Sundays follow a similar everyday schedule, you pursue on weekdays, and it's imperative to design your ends of the week ahead of time, particularly your dinners. A study led at Washington University and distributed in the diary Obesity, found that adjustments in timetable, dinners, and way of life practices on ends of the week were sufficient to cause weight put on or hinder weight reduction for the whole week. Numerous individuals can't make sense of for what reason they're not getting results when it appears as though they invest a lot of exertion throughout the entire week.

The appropriate response is that two days of extravagance can fix five days of work. Making arrangements for Holidays, Birthdays, and Special Occasions Planning is likewise instrumental for exploring your way through occasions, birthday events, parties, and other unique events. I accept that these are events where it's superbly suitable to unwind and appreciate the food, family, and fun that are a piece of these unique occasions. This doesn't mean overeating yourself or tossing all alerts to the breeze. Stay away from all-or-none reasoning. You don't need to pick between getting a charge out of the special seasons or remaining lean and solid—you can pick both.

Occasions and other get-togethers can undoubtedly be worked into your 10 percent consistency rule. Be that as it may, when you focus on 90 percent consistency, respect your guarantee to yourself. A typical example, particularly every November and December, is the "I'll start when" mentality. For reasons unknown, three occasions—Thanksgiving, Christmas, and New Year's—some way or another convert into about a month and a half of relentless dietary destruction. It's imperative to place this in a legitimate viewpoint. It's extremely just three days you need to manage.

Truth be told, it's just a couple of suppers. Appreciate the occasion food with some restraint. The remainder of the period it's preparation and nutritious eating, not surprisingly. If you discover yourself saying, "I'll start when I move beyond the special seasons," be cautious, since that sort of reasoning typically reaches out a long ways past January 1, and you'll generally be hoping to begin when conditions are perfect. They never are. Making arrangements for Vacations and Travel Just on the grounds that you're voyaging doesn't mean you can't pursue your ordinary food and preparing routine. You invest a lot of energy arranging the flight, the vehicle rental, the lodging, and different subtleties of your excursion, why not prepare and food?

Here's the absolute most dominant method I've at any point utilized for health and wellness: about each time

I travel, I set an objective to return home fit as a fiddle than when I left. Here are the means by which to do it:

- Get lodging with a kitchen. Numerous inn networks offer rooms with a full kitchen. Or then again attempt transient loft or condominium rentals. Search the Internet, and you might be amazed at the sort of cabin accessible and now and then at preferable costs over inns.
- Go food shopping following checking in. Subsequent to checking in, make a straight shot to the neighborhood supermarket, shopping list close by. Any place you are on the planet, If you have a kitchen and a well-loaded icebox, your supper arranging and food readiness is very little, not quite the same as when you're home.
- Check the neighborhood eatery menus ahead of time. When you travel, almost certainly, you'll have more café suppers than expected. Utilize all the eatery arranging techniques you adapted before

and consistently ponder what you'll eat each time you eat out.

- Prepare various types of foods and pack healthy snacks for drives, flights, and day trips. For long flights and drives, nothing beats convenient dinners and tidbits that you can convey with you. You can figure out how to make a variety of compact foods, including various kinds of cereal flapjacks, solid burgers, and sound sandwiches. Traveling, flying, or driving is never a reason for poor eating.

- Work out your exercise plan for advance. Continue utilizing your time organizer or timetable book in any event, when you're away from home. Continuously work from a composed arrangement.

- Pick your training area ahead of time. You can do bodyweight practices directly in your lodging. If you like, utilize the Internet to find a rec center before your outing. Bring ahead of time and inquire as to whether there is day by day or week after week rates. Inquire as to whether your inn has an exercise center or an alliance with a nearby fitness center.

In case you're an individual from an exercise center in your neighborhood, to check whether they are associated with different clubs around the nation. Make physical diversion part of your sightseeing plans. On one ongoing excursion, I spent a whole day climbing on the slopes of a wonderful national park. On another, I leased a bicycle and rode for miles along a beachside way. I've additionally seen other individuals, a significant number of them unfit, tooling around outside on those high-quality bikes. Which would you pick?

THE SUREFIRE WAY TO IMPLEMENT NEW HABITS AND LIFESTYLE CHANGES

There's no chance to get around it—to handle an issue like a muscle to fat ratio, which has such a large number of causes, you should make changes in each aspect of your life. You need to eat better, train reliably, deal with your feelings, change your reasoning, get the help you need, and set up everything together into a solid way of life. In any case, there's extraordinary power in organizing and focusing on the absolute most significant errand at some random time.

Numerous individuals attempt to do excessively, too early. The amazingly roused sorts may pull it off, yet the vast majority who make a plunge and roll out clearing improvements at the same time only dissipate their center, diffuse their endeavors, and end up with a lower achievement rate over the long haul. Another habit, as a rule, takes around twenty-one sequential days to shape. If you center around each essential objective or conduct change in turn, while keeping everything else in a holding design, you can shape seventeen new habits in a year.

With this methodology, one year from now, you will be such a changed individual, you'll need a telescope to think back to where you began. Locate your greatest restricting imperative, adhere to the 80-20 principle, and utilize the progressive system way to deal with picking the most sensible spots to begin. Every individual has one of a kind qualities and shortcomings, so you'll need to painstakingly pick which territories you need to organize and concentrate on first. Here's one case of how the initial six habit changes may play out.

1. Hit the sack at ten to eleven p.m. sharp, so you get seven to eight hours of value rest.
2. Take up yoga, contemplation, or unwinding activities to help lessen pressure.
3. Start having breakfast each day, which you may have skipped regularly. Attempt regular oats, blueberries, and an egg-white scramble with one entire omega-3 egg.
4. Exchange the leg "conditioning" practices you were accomplishing for nothing weight squats and deadlifts.

5. Quit drinking liquor or lessen to one to two beverages a few times per week.
6. Quit drinking pop and change to water or unsweetened green tea as your essential refreshments.

CHAPTER FOUR - PLANNING, ORGANIZING, AND IMPLEMENTING

If we gave your fitness and health habits an unexpected assessment today, what might be the prognosis? Be sincere. Would your eating routine be a critical condition, in critical need of crisis treatment? Would your training program need a bit of fixing up to a great extent? Do you, at any point, have an organized training program? What about your lifestyle? Is your body enduring the impacts generally late nights, liquor use, or significant levels of stress?

Notwithstanding your current physical condition, the absolute quickest method to improve your outcomes is by planning and prioritizing. Your central goal is to recognize which regions throughout your life need prompt consideration and afterward sort out the entirety of your exercises around those needs.

By following the recipe, you'll learn in this chapter, how you could go from a total stop to pedal to the metal and really show signs of improvement brings about less time. 80-20: The Magic Formula for Achieving More by Doing Less There's presumably no better method to set needs and increase your energy than observing the 80-20 rule.

It was first discovered in 1897 by Vilfredo Pareto, an Italian business analyst who saw a striking lopsidedness in the circulation of riches. He found that 20 percent of the populace had 80 percent of the cash and resources. In wellness, the 80-20 guideline is nonsensical. You may expect that all aspects of your preparation and food would have around similar importance. Subsequently, you, as a rule, treat every viewpoint similarly. Be that as it may, the 80-20 principle applied to fitness and wellness says that 20 percent of your food, planning, and habits will create 80 percent of the adjustments in your body.

Understanding this guideline can be unpleasant from the outset since you'll understand that the vast majority of what you were doing each day created almost no outcomes. You may wind up feeling like the proverbial gerbil on the wheel—lots of action, yet going nowhere fast. Then again, it's a significant disclosure since it implies that it's completely conceivable to get more comes about because of doing less. When you see how to utilize this to further your potential benefit by actualizing the standard, it's a groundbreaking change in perspective. You understand that you don't need to perspire the little stuff, so in that sense, it's freeing. Your frame of mind turns out to be progressively loose, and the entire undertaking is less upsetting because you quit stressing over each modest detail.

Applying the 80-20 guideline is a procedure of recognizing needs and concentrating more on those and less on everything else. It's the embodiment of working savvy. There are two different ways to apply the 80-20 standard:

1. Invest additional time and vitality on the imperative few (the 20 percent).

2. Invest less time and vitality on the unimportant many (the 80 percent).

The million-dollar question is, how would you know the contrast between the significant needs and the paltry subtleties? What are the 20 percent of exercises that are creating most of your outcomes? Finding and Eliminating Bottlenecks Think of the way to your ideal weight and perfect body as a gigantic multilane expressway. Then envision there's something blocking at least one of the paths. As autos must converge to the other side to press through a restricted passageway, a gag point is made, making traffic back up for miles, hindering your movement time or in any event, carrying you to a stand-still. Any individual who has ever been trapped in rush hour gridlock in Los Angeles or Chicago can identify with this since turnpike bottlenecks in those urban areas cause 25 to 27 million hours of the individual to delay each year.

Unnecessary delays likewise happen in your fitness venture since at least one significant path of progress is blocked. Coaches regularly whine about their customers demolishing all their difficult work in the exercise center because even as well as can't be expected to make up for a lousy eating routine. One change in your regular lifestyle routine, for example, lack of sleep, poor decisions in cafés, or end of the week gorging can demolish a whole seven day stretch of smart dieting.

A solitary restricting conviction, negative frame of mind, or enthusiastic issue can attack all that you do. Other basic limitations incorporate poor travel habits, skipping breakfast, passionate eating, hitting the bottle hard, poor practice structure, wasteful practice projects, and irregularity in any part of your sustenance or preparing. Requirements can either be heavily influenced by you (inside) or out of your control (outer). For the most part, you'll find that the greatest requirements are interior. As Pogo said, "We have met the enemy, and he is us." If you're not gaining ground toward your objective, there's quite often one significant requirement obstructing your way, and you quite often have authority over it. When you separate and get rid of it, your advancement begins to move through again at the most extreme conceivable speed.

Your body's shape and size will begin changing so quickly it's practically alarming. A basic question or two can assist flush with excursion the significant restricting imperative: What one snag is keeping down your advancement in each other territory? What one deadly defect has been keeping you from arriving at your objective? When you've bound the limitation, your need is to pour most of your vitality into settling that one major issue.

THE HIERARCHY OF NUTRITION

One of the ideal approaches to organize is by utilizing the chain of command approach. Abraham Maslow's progressive system of necessities, a mental hypothesis of inspiration, was one of the most celebrated chains of command. Shown as a pyramid, basic physiological needs, for example, food, water, and rest framed the biggest part at the base, and regard or self-realization needs, for example, accomplishment and imagination were the littler pieces stacked on top. As indicated by Maslow's chain of command, If the most fundamental life needs aren't satisfied, then they should become quick needs. Just when the basic endurance needs have been met can the higher needs be sought after. This pecking order idea is amazingly useful when you apply it to your preparation and sustenance. More than forty supplements are fundamental for your wellbeing, to give vitality, fabricate or fix body tissues, and perform different substantial capacities.

A caloric deficiency is a fundamental prerequisite for fat misfortune, however outrageous and delayed starvation eats fewer carbs to reduce your metabolic rate. Caloric hardship additionally makes it hard to get the various basics. Food is fuel, and you need to top off the gas tank each day If you need to go anyplace. Are you getting enough fuel? Basic amino acids. Protein is seemingly the most significant macronutrient when you're concentrating on fat misfortune. Protein causes you to clutch lean tissue while you're in a caloric deficiency, and it even smothers your hunger. Basic amino acids, which are the basic structures of protein, can't be made by your body, so you should get them from your food. Are you eating a lean protein with every supper and meeting your day by day protein necessities? Fundamental unsaturated fats. Essential unsaturated fats are imperatively significant for cardiovascular wellbeing and various body capacities, including consuming fat. Like basic amino, the essential unsaturated fats can't be integrated into your body and should be gotten from your food. Is it true that you include solid fat sources, for example, salmon consistently? Essential nutrients and minerals. Nutrients and minerals are natural or inorganic mixes vital for the legitimate working of your body. They're basic because your body can't make them or can't make them in sufficient amounts, so you should get them from your food. Organic cereals, fruits, and vegetables are among the most extravagant wellsprings of these micronutrients. Are you eating them reliably consistently? Water. Your body is, for the most part, water. Water is essential to the point that without it, you'd pass on in merely days. Indeed, even mellow parchedness diminishes physical execution. Satisfactory water admission is likewise important to consume fat, ideally.

These are the essentials that must frame the establishment of your pyramid. There are numerous minor subtleties that can take your sustenance to a more elevated level. In any case, If you understand you're inadequate in any of the basic pieces, that is the place your needs should go. Allude back to Chapter Six and the ten food rules to be certain your essential needs are met, to the exclusion of everything else. The Hierarchy of Training The primary essential of preparing is that you are preparing. Any preparation is superior to no preparation. Numerous individuals go through a long time examining preparing methods, yet never begin. Numerous individuals, particularly ladies, are reluctant to lift loads. Yet, weight preparation is a higher priority than vigorous preparation. Weight preparation can give cardiovascular medical advantages, yet heart stimulating exercise can't give quality or solid advancement benefits. Your selection of activities ought to likewise be organized, utilizing a chain of command of significance. All activities are not made equivalent. Continuously make the compound free-weight activities, for example, squats, thrusts, deadlifts, lines, and presses your first need.

The disconnection works out, for example, twists, triceps augmentations, and calf raises, are useful yet less significant, and accordingly, put rearward in the exercise. In case you're at any point in a hurry and need to abbreviate your exercises, drop these detail practices first, and consistently keep the significant developments. Most machines, except for certain link works out, take lower need than freeloads. If your lower body exercise comprises of leg expansions, leg twists, inward thigh machine, and butt blaster machine, you have to take care of your needs. Start hunching down and deadlifting. You'll get progressively out of those two free weight practices than every one of the four of the machines joined. Cardio is lower on the activity chain of importance than weight preparing, yet significant in any case. The perfect program contains weight preparation and cardio preparation.

Cardio gives its very own one of a kind wellbeing and wellness advantages and expands your all-out calories consumed. Similarly, as with weight training works out, the kind of cardio ought to likewise be organized. Try not to pass judgment on a cardio exercise dependent on time alone. A twenty-to thirty-minute cardio exercise could consume the same number of calories as an hour-long exercise. The thing that matters is a force. If you're healthy, fit, and have no orthopedic or therapeutic issues, then extraordinary cardio goes higher on the chain of importance, particularly if time proficiency is essential to you.

TRY NOT TO WASTE TIME

If 20 percent of your activities produce most of your outcomes, then by definition, 80 percent of your activities produce the minority of your outcomes and are generally insignificant. Worrying over details is the deadly problem in a large number of individuals' fat-loss goals.

A few people misconstrue the 80-20 decision to imply that nearly all that they're doing is useless. While that is not a long way from reality now and again, it's not so much exact. The 80 percent essentially speaks to bring down worth exercises. In case you're an aggressive competitor, propelled student, or refined calorie counter who has just aced every one of the basics and essentials, the subtleties matter. A great deal. Another significant achievement guideline is known as the triumphant edge hypothesis, which expresses that everything aides or damages, nothing is nonpartisan. This is particularly significant in sports, business, or aggressive undertakings, where the smallest edge tallies.

Do subtleties make a difference? Approach an Olympic swimmer for whom the distinction between a gold and a silver award was one-hundredth of a second. Ask the sprinter who set forth and missed the decorations by a tenth of a second. If you're an expert competitor, then apparently unimportant subtleties, arranging, and execution are the distinction between leaving a mark on the world and being a spectator.

- Everything matters. Everything tallies.

A little 100-calorie-per-day awkwardness in vitality—that is around four chocolate gulps from the sweet snack at work—could make you fat If you kept it up for a long enough timeframe and everything else stayed equivalent. The 80-20 standard doesn't infer that subtleties don't make a difference. It says you don't stress over the subtleties until you've aced the essentials. As Goethe stated, "The things that issue the most should never be helpless before things that issue the least."

- Always Have a Plan—

Never Wing It Imagine strolling by a building site and soliciting one from the laborers, "Hello, what are you all structure?" A specialist answers, "I have no clue." I wager you've never heard a wonder such as this since beginning to manufacture something without an arrangement would be senseless. In any case, did you ever think what it's just as senseless to go to a rec center, go shopping for food, or even take a seat during supper without an objective and composed outline for your sustenance and preparing? I once heard a statement from persuasive orator Jim Rohn that changed my reasoning for eternity. He stated, "Never start your day until you finish it." from the start, it seemed like a puzzle. How are you expected to complete your prior day you start it? Then the light went on, and I understood that he was talking about arranging before acting. The sensible augmentations are, never start your week until you've completed it, never start your month until you've completed it, and never start your year until you've completed it. Activity without arranging is perhaps the greatest reason for disappointment. Arranging requires genuine ideas and exertion. It requires a peaceful, centered time with a pen and paper or PC, frequently with a mentor or accomplice. Proficiency specialists state that consistently spent in arranging and arrangement will spare you ten minutes in execution.

When you apply this basic arranging idea to your sustenance, preparing, and way of life, the outcomes will stun you. Better results and increasingly productive utilization of time aren't the main benefits. Feeling ill-equipped or capricious makes tension and stress. That makes arranging and arrangement an amazing pressure reducer and certainty developer.

- **Arranging and Organizing Around Priorities**

Start each day, week, month, and year on paper. Continuously work from a list, plan, or timetable.

Compose a list of objectives, a list of day by day activity steps, an everyday plan, a week by week plan, a composed supper plan, a composed shopping list, and a composed preparing plan. Make need records, not plan for the day. Need records center around the imperative few. The plan for the day is generally jumbled with the minor many. The arranging procedure starts with an objective setting since every one of your exercises must be sorted out around your high-need objectives and wanted a new way of life habits. When your objectives are recorded as a hard copy, apply 80-20 reasoning. What is the one wellbeing, wellness, or body-weight objective that would have the greatest effect in your life? If you accomplished it in the following twelve weeks? Organize that objective by composing it on a card, conveying it with you wherever you go, and perusing it regularly.

- Take a look at every one of the five Body Fat Solution standards—

Mental training, cardio training, quality training, food, and social help. In every one of these classes, what is the one most elevated need objective or activity step that will have the greatest effect in your life? Make your week after week calendar and everyday activity plan around these needs. Every day and Weekly Scheduling Do you make meetings with your primary care physician? What about your dental specialist? Your bookkeeper? Your beautician? What about your life partner—do you plan a period and a day for dates? (Neighborly tip: If you don't, leave visas are impending.) If you make arrangements for everything else in your life, for what reason would you leave your preparation for whatever pieces of time happen to be leftover every day? Prepare to have your mind blown. There never is whenever left finished. Strangely, your schedule will consistently top off each day except if you set needs and calendar squares of time for what's generally critical to you. You can begin the arranging procedure with only a pen and a clean sheet of paper.

I prescribe putting resources into an arrangement book or time organizer.

Planning every week ahead of time is simple since you, as of now, might suspect and arrange your life on a week by week premise. You'll additionally be setting body-weight and body composition objectives and outlining your advancement on a week after week premise, making seven days the ideal square of time for arranging your preparation and food. I propose composing your week after week preparing plan into your time organizer each Sunday evening for the up and coming week. Then each prior night hitting the hay, survey your timetable, and set everyday objectives and needs for the following day.

CHAPTER FIVE: EATING OUT, STRATEGIES FOR DEALING WITH EMOTIONAL EATING OUTSIDE YOUR HOME

With our fast-paced ways of life, I think individuals now and then eat out more than they eat at home. Eatery and inexpensive food eateries, buffet meals, get-togethers, occasion meals, huge family social occasions, and excursion dinners can become uncommon difficulties for the greater part of us. Why? There are numerous reasons. When we eat out, we see that since we are not responsible for ingredients, arrangement, or in small sizes, "feasting out" signifies "getting out" or deserting our food plan. We may get confounded or feel vanquished by the number of decisions we should make when we destroy from home. Lastly, we may make presumptions about what is fitting conduct when we're eating out or even give ourselves authorization to binge.

A few people have not many challenges with eating out, yet they may battle with eating plans at home. Still, other individuals find that they are in charge when they eat at home, yet a gathering or eating out can be shocking for their eating plans.

Regularly we don't recollect every one of the things that work for us in a period of tumult, when feelings are running high, or when our quick paced world stretches us as far as possible. Know about oneself talk at that time. What are you letting yourself know? Is it accurate to say that you are looking into effective techniques or feeling despair on account of negative considerations? Decide to compose what works in the diary, utilize the diary, and keep mindful and change your self-talk. Work on that self-talk and alter territories of concern. Take 20 seconds to allude to the fitting segment—particularly this segment on eating out—and be set up for all outcomes with the goal that you can stay in charge and be fruitful.

Have an arrangement all set in your mind before you break the flow from your home meal plan? More than once, we have said, "To hell with the arrangement, I'll simply begin once again on Monday" isn't an alternative—and it is anything but a sensible methodology. You can deal with every one of your difficulties through mindfulness and arranging! In North America, the cafe experience is frequently appraised on the measure of food in singular servings. The pattern has been that the normal client will gripe whenever served a sensible portion, is by all accounts dependent on the nature of the food, but on the amount of food on individual plates. You have to prepare when you eat out in eateries. When placing an order, request a smaller part or a half-portion. Lots of eateries will readily do this. If the eatery doesn't agree, request a "take out" compartment to accompany your dinner.

This gives you the chance of passing judgment on your own part size and putting what you won't eat at that feast in the holder to bring home. Do this before you dive into the supper, and you will find that you most likely have enough in your holder for another dinner!

The reward: you won't be enticed to binge. A few eateries will guarantee that they don't have littler divides as a choice. However, they will furnish a plate with less food on it—in spite of the fact that they will charge you the maximum. This is really a sensible choice. If you eat the bigger feast, what is the genuine cost would you say you are paying regarding feelings, blame, fault, or disgrace? Is it justified, despite all the trouble to forfeit smart dieting, trouble your association with food, and endanger your associations with the ones you love?

Here is a list of systems I have discovered supportive when advising individuals about feasting out concerns and difficulties:

• Call the café early and have the menu faxed to you with the goal that you can choose what to arrange early that accommodates your eating plan.

• Pre-order your food to guarantee achievement If you are truly not certain about your capacity to arrange astutely before other individuals.

- Ask your host if it is OK to arrange first, so you are not enticed by what others are requesting.

- When you request, ask how things are readied. Inquire as to whether your request can be broiled or poached rather than fried.

- Order broiled veggies with your supper rather than pasta or pureed potatoes with sauce.

- Be cognizant with regards to requesting food with flavors, cream sauces, or sauces when all is said in done. Request them as an afterthought, so you can control the sum you expend. Simply dunk your fork into the sauce for enhancing as you take a snack of food.

- Be mindful of requesting food that accompanies serving of mixed greens dressings, nuts, high sodium meats, cheeses, bread 3D squares, nacho platters, olives, and guacamole. Request serving of mixed greens dressings as an afterthought—dunk your fork in them for enhancing as opposed to pouring them on your plate of mixed greens.

• Offer to part a supper with a friend if it is suitable. Approach your server to bring for another side plate with the goal that you can partition the dinner into two segments. Cafés are frequently glad.

• Ask the server before-hand to carry your plate when you are finished.

• When you are finished eating, place your blade and fork on your plate. Treat your palate like a clock: place the knife and fork together with handles at 5 o'clock, indicating 10 o'clock. Push the plate only a couple of inches from you with your thumbs on the edge of the plate to flag you are finished. If you have been utilizing a paper napkin, place it over your plate. (Legitimate behavior implies that you would not do this with fabric napkins; they ought to just be set on the table close to your plate.) These are signed to your server that you are done with your supper.

- If you decide not to eat the full segments you have been served, inquire as to whether you can have the rest of go.

FAST FOOD

Normally fast-food eateries serve foods that are high in fat, sugar, sodium, and starches. Late drifts in good dieting have incited some fast-food chains to make some solid decisions. Anyway, those things are not as well known, in some cases, sit on the rack for broadened timeframes, some of the time turn sour, and very regularly are immediately supplanted in the menu. Fast food ordinarily keeps to things that are prevalent and sell reliably, for example, high-fat substance burgers, fries, and carbonated refreshments stacked with sugar.

Fast food eateries have additionally experienced seen esteem being in the amount of their food. "Super-sized" suppers can be twofold or even triple the segments of fat, sugar, and sodium that we regularly devour in a whole day! If you decide to go to a fast-food eatery, plan to go to one where you will use sound judgment. One methodology is to arrange a children's feast to exploit the littler size; give the toy to the children. Look on the web and become more acquainted with a few fast food menus, so you know the rates and dietary benefits of their things and can make sense of what will work best for you early — that way, you are set up with a strategy.

Think about all the squandered vitality related to decision making and the squandered vitality if you don't settle on informed choices. The outcomes in your self-talk could be: blame, thrashing on yourself, disgrace, and emotions of loss of control. These emotions could ruin the entire occasion, in addition to influence your determination to keep up your good dieting arrangement. Relax! Eating fast food is unavoidable—so why not make it pleasant and keen! Settle on shrewd decisions. Select fast food suppers that will fit into your day by day eating plan, and keep to your objectives.

This might be simpler than it sounds if you recall thoughts regarding balance. For instance, envision that you enable yourself to have one little request of fries with a broiled chicken burger, mayo as an afterthought, with juice or water to drink. Gradually eat each fry in turn, tasting each snack, appreciating the supper. Understand that you don't need to complete the fries, realizing you are content with just having 6–8 pieces. Settle on a choice that the remainder of the fries is not worth going short on different foods later in the day. Acknowledge that, however, a couple is delicious, they are oily and too salty to even think about eating the whole bit. You realize that eating every one of them may give you an annoyed stomach, and you choose it's not justified, despite any potential benefits to eat them all. Poise implies you decide to be content as you pursue your arrangement and feel glad for yourself. You've put your breathing device on first:

you are dealing with yourself and breathing simpler about your association with food.

Well-Being "It will be awful! I don't have the foggiest idea of what to request to keep on my arrangement!" That is the way it will be. That is the thing that you have let yourself know, in this way you will make it so. Instead, you may state, "I will set myself up early, find out about my decisions, and settle on the best choice for my well-being." That is the thing that you will probably do.

BUFFETS

The scandalous buffet is regularly charged as "Everything YOU CAN EAT!" as though this were the objective of buffet feasting. Some dread the buffet table; some adoration it! Regardless of which side you are on, the visual effect of the buffet spread is some of the time overwhelming. The primary thought that strikes a chord concerning decisions was—what decisions are to be made, yet what are the best worth choices. A few people need to get their cash value. Typically the last decision to be made is, "The thing that on this buffet table is solid and fits into my eating plan?" Buffets sensibly connect with us in a great deal of self-talk because there are such a significant number of decisions to be made about such a large number of enticing dishes.

Self-talk may be very surprising for every individual, except it, regularly comes as a test to our feeling of decency. It doesn't need to be. If you are vexed about the value contrasted with the amount of food you intend to devour, who truly pays? It is safe to say that you are practical or sharp? Examine what is happening in your mind? About this theme, yet be progressively mindful of what you are informing yourself regarding food. Again and again, we have negative self-talk! Consider this. I did when I directed individuals. I would believe that it has cost a few people—in one year alone—3300 dollars to shed 45 pounds. I needed to inquire as to whether they were going to pass up being affected by their negative discussion about their association with food.

They had a decision to make. Is it safe to say that they would get every piece of significant worth from an eatery or buffet supper by devouring as much as they could, or would they say they would connect an incentive to the nature of their feasting out understanding? I would regularly transcend their protests and legitimizations by soliciting, "Shouldn't something be said about the cost of your well-being?" If buffets alarm you, don't go to one until you are alright with picking the correct foods and eating as indicated by your eating plan. Cost is extra; accept that you are paying for the experience, not the amount you can destroy or truck.

Here are a few methodologies for eating out at a buffet:

- If it is a cooperative choice to go to a buffet, and you are awkward with that decision, inquire as to whether anybody minds heading off to someplace else. If you feel bolstered, disclose that to the individuals in your gathering.

- Ask If you could meet them at the eatery after they eat. Or then again state that you are tied up to that point, and you will seek an espresso after.
- If you wind up heading off to the smorgasbord café, request a menu as opposed to picking the smorgasbord alternative. Feel certain the creation of this great decision and maintaining a strategic distance from the buffet table.
- Ask to be situated far away from the smorgasbord. If the smorgasbord is in somebody's home, sit far away from the smorgasbord table.
- If you decide to participate in the smorgasbord, study the spread for savvy decisions and furthermore for thoughts that will advance your prosperity. Adhere to your arrangement.
- Tell yourself that the foods on a smorgasbord table consistently look obviously superior to the taste. In reality, this is likely obvious because the foods are

set up in enormous amounts and kept warm or cold for quite a long time as opposed to being readied new for singular plates.

- Choose a littler plate If you can. If a littler plate isn't accessible, then remain inside the inward ring of the supper plate and don't put any food past that edge.
- Have a little soup to begin or an enormous serving of mixed greens.
- Have only a spot of what you might want to attempt. When you place the food tests on your plate, orchestrate it with the goal that foods don't contact one another.
- Take your time. Plunk down and make the most of your food. Taste each chomp; appreciate the organization.
- Have an organic product for dessert.
- Share a sugary pastry. If you should, however, have only a couple of snacks. Appreciate them. Enjoy the flavors. Enable yourself to have the taste without overindulging.

- When you are finished eating, place your blade and fork on the plate and cover your plate with your paper napkin. Move the plate away from you two or three inches. This flag you are done eating and a server can expel your plate.
- Resist the compulsion to return to the table for quite a long time." "Be straightforward with yourself about your eating design and be in charge. Relax!

GET-TOGETHERS

In many societies, numerous get-togethers are associated with foods. In your home, at work, and around your Friends, you may feel responsible for your food utilization. However, get-togethers may show an entire diverse arrangement of difficulties for you. Weddings, organization feasts, mixed drink parties, potlucks, retirement festivities, leaving parties, political meetings, craftsmanship opening gatherings, and church picnics are only a couple of instances of get-togethers that frequently serve food. The greatest test is that the food is generally free! My most exceedingly terrible time is "free" food at a gathering, meeting, or at another person's home.

As I examine the food table, I consider new plans, new food thoughts, food sources I don't typically have close by or don't ordinarily eat because they are on my "dangerous foods" list. Like such a significant number of individuals, when I'm in this circumstance, my first thought is that I should top off with free food. I am mindful that in my school years, this demeanor helped me to increase 15 additional pounds. This is such a notable marvel in new undergrads in Canada and the States that it is regularly alluded to as the "Green bean Fifteen"! I presently realize that "getting my fill" appeared in my midriff! Presently, as a grown-up, I am mindful that at a get-together, I can decide to have one taste of a solitary food thing and be fulfilled. I have figured out how to move my spotlight and rather focus on the event, the individuals, and the social parts of the occasion as opposed to on the food.

Here are some more methodologies that can assist you with concentrating on the occasion and not the food:

- Plan your day when you realize you will go out later. Pack your lunch and snacks prior in the day. Else you will be eager to such an extent that you will try too hard when you get to the occasion.
- Compensate for an event that you realize will be focused on food: plan additional activity and equalization out your everyday food admission.
- Ask what will be served, so you realize how to prepare it in time.
- Plan to eat with some restraint and alter your bits as needs are. Pick solid foods.
- If you should have a sweet pastry, select one that is your least most loved, so you do not eat a lot of it.
- Ask your host or leader If you may to carry a dish to the occasion—make it something that you can fit into your eating plan.
- Do you have a help individual with you? Tell that help individual early about any food or eating

difficulties you hope to experience. Discussion about the help you need.

- Show up to the occasion later to maintain a strategic distance from the tidbits. Eat before you go.
- Pre-divide your plate with foods that fit your arrangement and just eat what is on your plate to abstain from picking.
- Focus on the non-food themes and on different visitors.
- Keep a solid beverage in your grasp consistently; make it a full or half-full glass to guarantee nobody inquires as to whether you need a beverage.
- Keep a handbag, or a plate, cutlery, and a napkin in the other hand to shield you from snacking at the food or topping off your plate.
- Keep the discussion going as you avoid the table or the treats.
- Help the hosts by taking void plates or cups the kitchen to abstain from being enticed to snack at the food contributions.

Here are some close to home instances of procedures I use. As you probably are aware, I love chocolate brownies. However, if they have nuts in them, I am less inclined to eat them and enjoy them. Along these lines, If I have brownies on my very own occasion, I purchase ones with nuts in them. At Halloween, I get the chocolate bars that simply don't taste great to me, so I avoid them. A choice is to plan the get-together to occur at your home. Have a lot of sound options on the menu. Maybe you could get ready just what you know you to remain on track as opposed to having enticing foods on the menu that are not a piece of your arrangement. Plan to serve a few foods that you enable yourself to eat, so you don't feel denied.

If planning an occasion at your home is excessively unpleasant or is an over the top allurement with food planning, propose that another person have the occasion. Thoroughly consider it—what will be better for you? If you do have the occasion at your home, do you trust you can control things better? Make sense of this. Have an arrangement in any case. Here are some self-disclosure journaling questions that may assist you with seeing progressively about your association with food at get-togethers.

HOLIDAYS AND FAMILY FESTIVITIES

Holidays can be a challenge for us all. There is at any rate one holiday for each month in America—and maybe more If we incorporate strict and ethnic occasions. For some families, occasions, for example, weddings, commemorations, birthday events, and reunions are events celebrated with food. Thus, with regards to eating out, at any rate once per month, we have the chance to be tested in the good dieting division. Where do we start? You have to tune in to your positive self-talk, know, prepare, have techniques set up and inhale each day—or you could be in a tough situation. Possibly you sense that you are now in a tough situation. It's OK—take it each day in turn, and you can deal with these events. Your packed food schedule didn't occur without any forethought. Be caring to yourself and work through this diary; keep it with you and use it! Take the entirety of your systems for eating out and apply them to holiday and family festivities too.

Plan ahead and choose what you will do all together, not to try too hard. On the event, ensure you have a sample of everything If you wish. Simply don't surpass your everyday food consumption plan. Maybe you have a most loved occasion or family food. Appreciate it, however, balance it inside your day or choose to practice more to redress. Discover some help, focus on partition size, tune in to your self-talk, and change it if essential. Hold returning to mindfulness and your systems. Remind yourself about your objectives, why you need to be sound.

GET-AWAYS

Being away from home resembles eating out three times each day, so survey your techniques in this part, "Why You Eat." When you are on an excursion, utilize a meal plan that ensures you remain a similar weight, or to keep up your weight. Be savvy, healthy, be sound, and be effective! How and what would you be able to design? Here are some explicit get-away techniques to increase the ones we have just secured:

• Plan ahead and find out about the foods that are in your movement region.

• Be safe with foods! Counsel your nearby trip specialist and your well-being facility about risky foods in underdeveloped nations.

• On the street, bring a cooler and fill it with healthy food and snacks–organic product, squeeze, and hacked up veggies.

• When in an inn or motel, approach early for a kitchenette; inquire as to whether your room has a microwave and cooler.

• At your goal, go to prescribed nearby food markets for sound tidbits and feast ingredients.

- Ask if the kitchen in your inn, motel, or resort highlights solid menu options.

- Eat with some restraint.

EMOTIONALLY SUPPORTIVE NETWORKS: GETTING ENOUGH AIR

Having individuals who bolster you is significant with regard to your weight, the executives, and dealing with yourself. This emotionally supportive network gives positive consolation while simultaneously keeps you responsible. Here are a couple of general thoughts regarding how emotionally supportive networks work. Individuals in your care group ask how they can best help you in the challenges you face with eating and food. Bolster individuals don't chasten you or treat you gravely when you have had an awful food experience; rather, they tune in, offer proposals, and ask how they can help you later on.

On different occasions, you may require your care partners to be firmer with you than on different occasions. Be clear with them ahead of time that you depend on them to help you in specific manners and not in others—speak with them and reveal to them what you need. Together, you and your care partners can have any kind of effect. Try not to control your help individuals. They are there for you. I realize it can happen because I have done it—I've controlled somebody who was attempting to help me so as to get what I needed temporarily. Luckily it didn't work since I could have endangered my objectives to practice good eating habits.

Monitor what works for you to help. Every individual has an alternate approach, and every individual has various needs. Some like help to be conveyed delicately; however solidly, others acknowledge productive encounters, inspirational talk, and fervor. Still, others favor severe support. You choose what you need right now and be adaptable enough to transform it as your needs change.

SUPPORT FROM HOME

Specifically, our home support depends on the individuals who live with us and are generally acquainted with our needs and difficulties. If your emotionally supportive network is comprised of relatives or individuals who live with you and are not exactly alluring, it is imperative to at any rate chat with these individuals. Tell them how glad it would make you If you had somebody on your side to help you. If you have individuals who need to be on your help group, however, really are out to attack your prosperity, you might need to constrain your time with those individuals until you feel less enticed to bargain your arrangement and increasingly enabled to stay with it.

Maybe you live without anyone else. Who else could give home help? A few thoughts for help individuals who don't live with you however who know about your home life may be a nearby family member, a Friend or colleague, parent or kin, your neighbor, a rec center accomplice, your fitness coach or weight reduction advocate, or your chiropractor or specialist.

Here are a couple of ways your home emotionally supportive network can work successfully:

- When you are enticed to have foods that are not part of your program, food sources that you have distinguished as being hazardous, or If you figure you may start to gorge on food, your help people will be aware of those perils and inquire as to whether they can do or say whatever would assist you with moving beyond this scene. For instance, they may help with an interruption system to assist you with forgetting about food.
- When you feel enticed by foods, converse with your help individual immediately and request that the person in question help you. Try not to anticipate that that individual should think about

what you are thinking or police everything you might do.

- Ask your help individuals to move high-hazard foods to a zone you are ignorant of or is difficult for you to reach.
- Suggest that your care partners do not eat high-chance foods before you, or if nothing else inquire as to whether it OK to eat before you.
- Supporting individuals ought to be urged to inquire as to whether you need some rousing consolation to deal with your eating program. Maybe they could help you to remember your objective to eat well food, deal with your weight, and not feel caught or worried about your food decisions.

SUPPORT AT WORK

Do you have an emotionally supportive network at work? If you invest a great deal of energy at work, you will require support there similarly as you need at home. If you feel great doing as such, request that individuals at work assistance bolster your good dieting objectives. Work can be a hazardous situation if there are colleagues or individuals in your work environment who are not on a similar wavelength as you in attempting to practice good eating habits.

Some colleagues or Friends will need you to eat as they do with the goal that they don't feel so terrible about what food and well-being decisions they are making. If so, enroll some collaborators to help you. Likely they likewise will perceive these as difficulties for themselves, and you may find that you will shape a common bolster group. With mindfulness, eagerness, procedures, positive self-talk, and a decent, emotionally supportive network, this could be your key to progress!

At work, your help individual or group is there for you. Like your help individuals at home, these supporters don't chasten you or hatred you when you have had a terrible involvement in food. Rather they ask how they can support you. They get you persuaded, keep you propelled, and cheer you on if that is the thing that you need. They remind you how significant your objectives are.

When you are going to eat something that isn't in the arrangement and is unfortunate, speaks with your help individuals: request that they help you, don't simply accept it's their accountability to comprehend what is happening in your mind. Your help individual would then be able to assist you with maintaining a strategic distance from the circumstance. Maybe they will help with one of your interruptions to get you away from food. Perhaps they will help by moving high-chance foods to a territory out of your sight and reach. Your work bolsters individual or group will be delicate to eating high-hazard foods before you. They can investigate with you a few inspirations to keep to your arrangement and objectives to be successful.

If your emotionally supportive network at work is not exactly alluring, maybe it is essential in any event to converse with them. Tell them how glad it would make you If you had somebody on your side to help you. If you have an emotionally supportive network that is out to attack the entirety of your prosperity, you might need to constrain your time with those individuals until you feel progressively good about being around them in circumstances where enticing foods are being served. Keep occupied with work and ventures until you feel increasingly sure about this.

If there are no genuine help applicants in your work environment, attempt other people who could bolster where you work. Is there somebody that you believe works near your office? Is there somebody that you constantly see during noon? When you do discover some help in your workplace, monitor what works for you. Every individual has an alternate approach, and every individual has various needs. You choose what you need and change it to fit.

Here are a few methodologies that you and your work environment support group can do together to help one another:

- Keep occupied with your work. It is imperative to keep centered and abstain from pondering food.
- Plan in your snacks with your breaks; bring solid snacks and snacks from home.
- Always destroy from your work area.
- Drink water during the day and have your water bottle in every case full.
- Resist the impulse to keep desserts and snacks on or in your work area.
- Get up and stroll around If you are situated throughout the day!
- Challenge the workplace to choose progressively nutritious tidbits and suppers.
- Switch to more advantageous choices for office birthday, move, or retirement festivities—for instance, attempt a natural product flan as opposed to a chunk cake with thick icing.

- Ask if the sound tidbits can be placed in one organizer and less nutritious bites sorted out in another cabinet that you won't go into.
- Get the workplace roused to begin strolling at noon.
- Encourage others to pursue your habit for taking the stairs as opposed to the lift or lift.

If your working environment doesn't present specific difficulties—that is incredible—however, imagine a scenario in which you move to a new position in an alternate office or even to an alternate organization. You could wind up in an alternate working environment dynamic later on. I suggest that regardless, you answer the inquiries beneath in this diary, move a portion of those plans to your Journal, and afterward occasionally, particularly if your work environment changes, survey what is essential to you and what works. You may decide to impart a portion of these plans to your work environment bolster individual or people, or If you have framed a shared help group, you may jump at the chance to examine a portion of these thoughts together.

If they feel that it is sheltered to do as such, a few people will converse with the individual who is persistently pushing food and clarify that this conduct might be hazardous for others attempting to control their food consumption. To evade that individual, you can eat in an alternate zone, make outside lunch arrangements, or get things done outside the workplace. If an experience is unavoidable, consistently be lovely to the food pusher. For instance, when I wound up in an office with an individual who was continually pushing food on others, I kept my plate loaded with solid food sources and pleasantly stated, "Not this time—I have something as of now."

Much the same as the systems you use at home, interruption strategies can be essential to assist you with enticing or testing foods and food circumstances at work. Contingent upon your particular work, you may have the option to fit a portion of these interruptions into your workday. Here are five classifications that may support you:

1. Things that should be possible rapidly during work:

- Take a restroom break. Enjoy your break early, and appreciate the snack you arranged.
- If you are responsible for reusing and need to clear the little containers, do it now.
- If you have to go to verify the mail or drop something in another office, do it now.

2. Busy exercises during work—things that will absolutely remove your psyche from food or occupy a ton of time:

- Engage in any venture that requires close scrupulousness.
- Set a motivation for your next gathering or review the minutes from the last gathering.
- Work on your yearly report.
- Contact customers.

3. Things you can do on breaks at work:

- Go for a walk.
- Walk the stairs.
- Run a task.
- Balance your checkbook.

4. Things that are unwinding during breaks:

- Take a breather outside.
- Go into the meeting room if it's empty and unwinds.
- File your nails.
- Go to your vehicle for a rest and have somebody call you in a short time after your break is finished.

5. Things you can do with others or with others around you:

- Plan the workplace softball match-up.
- Plan the staff BBQ.
- Organize the following office philanthropy occasion.

- Start an office book club, sports lottery, or class arrangement.

When you have a challenge with food and eating at work, choose which classification will fit into your work routine. Select one of the exercises to finish, and If you need more interruption, then proceed with choosing another action. You may find that you can consider just a couple of interruption classifications in view of the sort of work that you do. Maybe your classifications are, for the most part, fit to exercises that you can do during snacks or breaks. That is fine— simply record pragmatic interruption techniques that fit you and your work environment. If you telecommute, you will have some extraordinary interruption thoughts from those you would have in an increasingly traditional office circumstance. Whatever your work environment, if food and food circumstances are a test, be set up to plan your very own interruption classifications. This strategy works! You will occupy yourself from considering food so you can continue ahead with your work—and conceivably proceed onward to greater and better things.

FRIENDS AND SUPPORT

Friends can be an extraordinary help—or they can be an issue. A few Friends can be exceptionally strong, while different Friends can need you to remain unfortunate, so they have somebody to be undesirable with. Try not to confuse support with compassion. Try not to believe that by sharing food, you are getting support; you could wind up becoming involved with another person's pity party. That isn't the target. If you get great help from Friends and are a decent help to other people, you would be shocked how well you will do. I comprehend that there will be days that you won't give or get impeccable help, however, quiet yourself at the time and consider your self-talk.

Gain into power by utilizing your Distraction Techniques.

Remind yourself why it is imperative to be stay on course. Get support from Friends and, thus, be a mentor and an incredible model! If your emotionally supportive network is not exactly attractive, maybe it is significant in any event to converse with your Friends and let them realize how glad it would make you If you had somebody on your side to help you in arriving at your objectives. If you feel that your Friends may unknowingly or incidentally damage the entirety of your endeavors to control your food admission, you might need to constrain your time with them until you feel progressively great around circumstances where you might be enticed to surrender your program. Try not to control their Friends' help. They are there for you. More than family or work connections, Friends might be the most powerless to our controls on the grounds that, out of kinship, they need to satisfy us and not feel they have over-ventured the limits of good kinship.

There are uncommon difficulties in requesting that Friends bolster you—be delicate and know about them! Yet additionally know about the endowment of a Friend's help; it might be the most valuable blessing you claim or can give. Do you and Friends consistently assemble around food? When you are with Friends, keep occupied with exercises and activities that don't include food until you feel progressively sure of remaining in charge. Plan getting together after supper or for espresso. Make the most of your kinships, yet additionally, recall the agony related to eating undesirable as opposed to breathing simpler about your association with food. Keep your fellowships invigorating and steady!

CONCLUSION

Here are a couple of definite instances of techniques and indications to support you on your voyage to a healthy well being while successfully managing emotional eating:

- Unless you have a lot of weight to lose and you can't cope with the dress you have, hold on to purchase littler measured attire until you arrive at your objective.
- Alter some exemplary pieces you effectively possess until you accomplish your objective weight, or relying upon how a lot of weight you intend to lose, purchase just a couple of outfits to endure this progress time until you arrive at your objective.
- Get free of your bigger estimated apparel. Give the garments or put them in a recycled shop or transfer store. Get a portion of your garments there too—you may locate some awesome outfits there while you change to your objective weight!

- For inspiration, experience your wardrobe and compose your garments from the biggest size to the littlest size. Mess around with your storeroom as you progress through the sizes from enormous to little. Make certain vestments small objectives.

- Hang outfits that you are practically prepared to fit into before your room entryway, so you physically need to stroll past them in the first part of the day and night. These "objective outfits" will help you to remember what you are doing.

- Write notes containing positive self-talk and certifiable articulations. Stick them everywhere throughout the house to remind yourself about your objectives. Compose your objectives on the notes too.

- Wear marginally more tightly fitting garments to remind you all the time that you have to eat better to quit being awkward. Indeed, even go to the extraordinary of putting on a somewhat tight swimming outfit under your apparel for the day to keep you propelled. When you get too agreeable is the point at which you are bound to eat inaccurately. This is amusing works, however!

- Picture yourself 5 or 10 pounds lighter—or 20 pounds lighter! Go to the supermarket and buy a 5, 10, or 20-pound pack of potatoes and put them in a knapsack. If your back well-being will permit it, convey this potato-filled pack around for a day. Feel the help by the day's end when you remove that rucksack. See what shedding those pounds can feel like? Pounds not lost distinctly to be found once more—you've freed yourself of those pounds for good!

- Visualize yourself in your ideal weight, what will your body feel like at that point? Your body will feel extraordinary. Indeed, even 10 pounds has any kind of effect. Thus, eating great and doing activities will make you feel much improved. If you are keeping up your objective weight. Imagine your feeling of success as an individual who can smile at your relationship with food.

Motivation, amazing thoughts, positive energy, and a general feeling of well-being are the prizes of utilizing the Strategies and techniques outlined in this book. By what means will your apparel fit? What will it feel like to settle on healthy food choices? How empowering is it to feel that you are not just settling on savvy decisions with regards to food and eating You have just to envision yourself at your objective weight and realize that you are the creator of your own success story., yet that these are your decisions! Don't give up! Don't relent! I will be cheering and rooting for you!

CPSIA information can be obtained
at www.ICGtesting.com
Printed in the USA
LVHW081155200422
716646LV00014B/580